HEALTHY

LIVING

SORTED

Chris Walker

ChrisWalker1812@gmail.com

About the Author

Chris Walker was born in Bristol in 1945 on the day before VE day. Just ten months after the end of the war his family moved out of Bristol and settled for rural life in Wiltshire.

He moved back to Bristol in 1962 and found a job with a bank. He worked in various locations in the city, then London, and one brief spell in New York.

His long career in financial services involved a lot of sitting at desks, with no exercise. He developed a daily routine over the years consisting of morning and afternoon snacks (doughnuts were a favourite) and a full lunch, with little thought given to a healthy lifestyle.

In spite of this regime, his weight throughout his earlier working years remained fairly constant – that is until he stopped smoking in 2003. This event led to him putting on the pounds; in 2018 he decided this could not continue.

Something needed to be done. He started reading about how best to improve his overall health and achieve an acceptable weight. His studies led to this short book.

Now retired, he lives in Farnham, Surrey. He is married with three daughters and six grand-children.

This is his third publication.

Contents

Continued...

1

What's it all About?

In my research into how best to maintain a healthy weight and stay fit, I found considerable advice. This book is a summary of my findings.

I have collected ideas and suggestions from the various fads of the moment, from hearsay, and from advice offered by healthcare and medical professionals. This has led to an element of repetition in the following pages caused by some of the same points - good points - being made in different ways.

I apologise for this repetition but it is not necessarily a bad thing if the point being made is worthwhile. My experience is that if I read or hear about something more than once, I am more likely to remember it.

I am aware of some inconsistencies in advice, for
example the benefits or otherwise of cheese – an
excellent source of protein, calcium and some
vitamins but also high in calories, and fattening.
When I am in doubt with issues such as this, I try
to use a bit of common sense and make my own
judgement.

Over time, thoughts on what food is good and
what is bad conflict, so you might not agree with
all the points I make. Fair enough, we live in a
constantly changing world.

As you read some sections of the book, I can hear
you say 'I know all this', because at times that is
how I felt when carrying out my research. But
without doubt I need to be reminded on a regular
basis of the road that must be taken to achieve a
healthy lifestyle.

The text is spaced-out for an easy and quick read
but I do suggest you read the book slowly to
absorb and remember those bits you tend to
agree with. Feel free to ignore those bits with
which you disagree.

You will find no recipes here. There is an
inexhaustible supply of healthy recipe books out
there and the market really does not want me to
add to the pile (although I acknowledge I am

adding to the overload of books on healthy eating
and lifestyle…)

My intention is to try to explain the theory behind
how I am training my mind (albeit not always
with total success) to act in such a manner as to

Lose Excess Weight and Get Fit

Disclaimer: please note I am not a nutritionist,
nor a health professional in any way, but just a
guy interested in collating ideas and suggestions
on healthy living.

First, an overview. I call it *My Plan*.

2

My Plan

I never call *My Plan* a diet: that would be a sure
way to fail
It is more a natural way of living.

Some say - 'Eat less, Exercise more'
That makes sense, we've all heard it before
but it's much easier said than done.

I set myself easy ways to exercise;
Nothing too strenuous at first
Like finding an excuse to walk up the stairs.

With exercise, the more the merrier
although it can be a struggle
to maintain motivation
when lethargy steps in.
But maintain motivation I must.

Exercise is good, essential in fact
but is only part of *My Plan*
A sensible approach to food is also required.
'Everything in moderation, nothing in excess
Who said that first? *

I taught myself to stop smoking
Now I am teaching myself to control my weight;
but I admit I have lapses.

I do not set myself unachievable goals
I keep it simple; I keep it manageable.

I tell myself:
I am not an over-eater any more
that's all in the past
I am no longer that person.
Surely life without gluttony can't be all bad.

This is a change for life, not just a week, a month
or a year
but a permanent change in behaviour.

It can do wonders for self-esteem to be
rewarded with a great sense of achievement,
and to see those pounds melting away.

Socrates c 500 BC

Some think about getting external help
such as joining a slimming club.
That's great when it works
and if it's maintained,
but I am still trying to do it myself
and manage it myself.

And I try to follow that excellent piece of advice
from *Monty Python:*

Always Look on the Bright Side of Life

3

Ten thoughts on why I should stop unnecessary eating

And mentally how to do it

1. Am I actually hungry?

2. Overeating is a habit. Like smoking

3. I am going to stop an unpleasant habit

4. When tempted, I can have a glass of water, or a piece of fruit or veg. Or suck a mint

5. Or perhaps go for a short walk

6. I can distract myself with something in the
    environment. What's the weather doing?
    What's on telly tonight?

7. I should not need reminding about the health
    dangers of overeating

8. I will be just a little less embarrassed looking
    in the mirror

9. I think of the extra energy I will have to
    enjoy life more

10. It need not be such a big event; let's keep it
    simple and just do it

Some of these thoughts will be expanded later

4

I remind myself why getting my weight down to a sensible level is a Good Thing to Do

I will feel fitter and more comfortable

I will have more energy to be able to walk up the hill where I live without puffing and panting

My self-esteem will improve, I will feel better about myself

I am not a vain person, but my appearance, body-shape wise, should improve

I might even snore less and sleep better.

5

And I must remember what obesity can lead to…

Diabetes

Heart diseases

Strokes

Stomach and bowel ailments

Strain on the kidneys, especially from alcohol

In my case, I suffer from indigestion and heartburn which is worse when I am particularly overweight. This increases my risk of oesophagus cancer. Not good.

6

What about snacking?

Well, it's not a good thing but I have collected suggestions as to what to do when that between-meals hunger *(imagined or otherwise)* sets in:

Try to distract your mind, for example by saying to yourself, 'I'll come back to that thought in a minute'. And yes, sometimes the craving will go away

If not, drink a small glass of water as suggested earlier or a cup of herbal tea (without milk)

Try an apple or pear

A tomato, sliced carrot or a stick of celery

A small handful of unsalted nuts, preferably almonds

Or a slice of plain Ryvita, perhaps thinly spread
with Marmite if you like it (I love it)

Cleaning your teeth apparently works for some

If the weather is fine, go for that short walk and
take in the surroundings to divert your mind from
food.

. . . .

Perhaps this is a good place to emphasise the
health benefits gained by just simple walking.

These include:

Improved circulation

A boost to immunity

Relaxation of the brain

Improved memory

A lightening of your mood

Relief from stress

And not least a reduction in the risk of diabetes and heart disease.

My problem with snacking, and I suspect is shared with many others, is when watching TV in the evening.

Temptations arise and my thoughts stray to snacking – the cheese in the fridge, the biscuit tin, or the bar of chocolate I know is hidden in the cupboard.

At these times I try to imagine how I will feel in the morning if I lapse into scoffing comfort food – I know full well I will be disappointed and annoyed with myself.

Why take a backward step against my good intentions and waste my progress so far, for just a moment's pleasure?

. . . .

Time now to quote from a professional – Allen Carr, who encouraged millions of people to quit smoking with his bestselling book, *Easy Way to Stop Smoking*. I was one of the millions.

He later published a sister book, *The Easy Way to Lose Weight,* and a brief summary of Carr's mantra on controlling weight follows in the next chapter.

He believes in *training the mind.*

7

It's Attitude of Mind that Matters

Be positive and feel the excitement of what you might achieve

Over-eating is like any addiction, be it smoking, alcohol or drugs

Only eat if truly hungry, not if just thinking about it

Try not to snack between meals

Give priority to natural food

Avoid all junk food, processed food and refined food

Drink water in preference to other beverages

Train your mind to accept what you know is right

Create healthy meals but a word of warning – if these are unnecessarily complex and time consuming, you might not stick with your resolve

Just believe it need not be such a big deal.

………..…………

I recently asked a close friend if, like me, he usually enjoyed a drink before his evening meal and a glass (or two) of wine with the meal. He replied:
    'My default drink is water'

Made me reconsider my drinking habits…

So what's so special about water? Well, according to my research, these are some of the benefits gained by drinking just plain water:

Improved digestion

Help in preventing fatigue and can lead to
improved energy levels

An improvement in brain function

May relieve constipation

Improved skin complexion

Help in preventing headaches

All sounds good to me!

8

Media Contributions

Here follows tips and suggestions from a variety of newspaper and magazine articles, and some thoughts from myself; a generic summary albeit with some repetition of advice given elsewhere. But this collection of thoughts and ideas has helped me immeasurably.

Here goes:

To start, how do you know if you are clinically overweight, or just a bit on the plump size (apart from seeing your naked body in the mirror)?

One option is to measure your Body Mass Index (BMI). There is a formula for this but preferably, and much easier to use, is the BMI Calculator on the NHS website.

A reading of between 20 and 25 is Normal, below 20 is Underweight, over 25 is Overweight, over 30 is Obese and over 40 is Morbidly Obese.

When I first became concerned about my weight, my BMI was hovering around the 30 plus mark. Using the calculator today, my BMI has reduced to 26.1 – still overweight, but with a little more effort I can move down into the Normal range. I'm working on it.

Having said all this about BMI, many dietitians now believe the relationship between your waist and height is more significant. They reckon your waist measurement should be no more than half your height. My height is 180 cm but my waist is 96 cm, so I still have some way to go.

This formula is quite challenging but really important, because fat around the midriff risks damaging vital internal organs.

Enough about measuring the body; let's move on with suggestions relating to food:

If you have to snack, choose vegetables such as sliced carrot, pepper, mushroom, cucumber or a tomato

Or celery. It doesn't look like much but actually is rich in vitamins, minerals and antioxidants, has a low glycaemic index (good) and can help digestion. And it takes longer to chew – a good thing

An apple a day keeps the doctor away (a favourite expression from those days when GP's made regular house calls…)

Eat a small handful of nuts a day. Examples suggested are almonds (best), walnuts, pistachios or brazil nuts

Potatoes, white rice and pasta all raise blood sugar levels. A bad thing

Look for foods with low fat, low sugar content

Avoid all fatty and processed meats

No fried food, whether chicken, battered fish, chips or crisps

No sugary foods – biscuits, cakes, chocolate.

That's all very well but there are a lot of No's here and arguably too restrictive to be fully successful. Perhaps if read as 'reduce consumption of' might be more workable. It is of absolutely no use setting unattainable targets.

No peanuts, nor any salted nuts. It's not the salt itself that is fattening (although it can lead to increased blood pressure and water retention) but the addition of salt makes the nuts (more) addictive.

Occasionally skip a meal —a daytime fast can be very effective. In due course the body will start to use fat reserves for energy instead of using the missed meal. Any process that increasingly uses fat reserves in this way will – in time – force your body into a state of ketosis and you will lose weight.

This effect has led to the popular, but sometimes controversial, *Keto diet* and I have noticed in my local bookshop an ever-increasing supply of books covering the subject.

Quick-fire tips

Have an alcohol-free day at least once a week

Eat nothing after 7pm

Check calories, fat and sugar content using the 'traffic light' information on the packet – this can be a source of surprises

Drink water before a meal

Check portion sizes

Use a smaller plate

Small mouthfuls

And use smaller cutlery – child's cutlery, perhaps

Put cutlery down between each mouthful

Chew slowly and eat slowly to feel satiated sooner

Don't pile food on your fork/spoon for the next mouthful until your mouth is empty from the previous loading

Think for a moment before taking that second helping

Perhaps leave some food on the plate

 Stop before feeling full

What your mind wants is not always the same as
what your body needs

That's a lot about food.

. . . .

 Exercise is also very important but it's not
essential to join a gym. Too much money is
wasted on gym memberships that are not fully
utilised (if at all).

Walking up and down stairs, ironing and
vacuuming, gentle gardening, are all good forms
of exercise. Every little helps.

Weightlifting – not the extreme sport you might
see on Channel 5, but the exercise you can do at
home. Weight-lifting burns belly fat and builds
muscle.

A while ago, I bought a small set of weights
which ranged from lightweight to back-breaking.

I selected a set of medium weights which I use regularly and find this helpful in toning my body.

But I am careful not to over-do it so I will never be a *Charles Atlas* (remember him?), neither do I ever want to have such a body.

My aim is just to maintain a normal shape.

And finally for this chapter, a doctor in Bristol (Dr. Dowling, I believe) once suggested, to improve posture as much as to lose weight, watching TV standing up…

9

Alcohol and Other Thoughts

Alcohol is packed with sugar and calories but these are called 'empty calories', meaning calories are consumed without any benefit apart, of course, from that temporary 'feel good' factor

Alcohol can raise blood pressure and increase heart rate

No alcohol is healthy but according to reports, spirits are arguably a better bet than wine. Pre-mixed spirits are best avoided

But conversely, some medical professionals recommend a glass of whisky or brandy at bedtime to get a good night's sleep

Alcohol encourages the brain to think of food, stimulating appetite and creating a feeling of hunger, which is why fattening crisps and other snacks go so well with an aperitif

Drinking alcohol can derail dietary resolve so it's never going to be good for your weight

It helps not to leave the bottle on the table during the meal…

....

Foods high in cholesterol and saturated fat are not good, and include:

Dairy – full fat milk, cream, butter and cheese

Sausages, meat pies, bacon and all fatty meat

Biscuits, cakes, coconut and ice cream. I thought ice cream was not so bad until I read it is full of sugar, calories and additives

Takeaway food, especially Chinese, is full of fat, salt and sugar – leave it out

I love Danish pastries but a standard-sized one contains up to 400 calories

White meat is healthier than red meat

Protein is essential and should be included in every meal

Favourite healthy protein foods include chicken, fish, beans and nuts

And I love cheese, but…

A summary of good and bad food is included in the next chapter

. . . .

Now another refence to exercise:

Oxygen converts glucose into energy. It follows that modest or strenuous exercise leads to breathing more rapidly, drawing more oxygen into the body, therefore creating energy from the excess glucose in the body.

Major benefits of burning off glucose are an improvement in blood glucose readings and a reduction in weight.

In the next chapter I reproduce a chart, personal to me, listing examples of food divided into categories. Others might compile a slightly different list.

These groupings have helped me concentrate on healthier living although I have lapses, I am only human. But I'm getting fewer lapses than before.

10

There's Good Food – and Bad Food

Good food

Small portions

Fibrous foods, as fibre slows sugar absorption

At least five fruit and vegetable portions a day

Vegetable stir-fry's

Beans including baked beans

Butternut squash

Mushrooms, peppers and tomatoes

Onions, leeks, broccoli and garlic

Virtually all vegetables really, not forgetting your greens

Nuts, but not peanuts, and not salted

Oily fish such as salmon, sardines, tuna or mackerel – but no fried fish

Porridge oats

Muesli with no added sugar

Apples and pears

Dried apricots

Yogurt – live or bio is best

Eggs in moderation

Steak (small and lean)

Pork tenderloin

Green tea or just water

Root ginger infused in tea or grated into soups and other food

Apple cider vinegar (one tablespoon to four of water) before a meal can lead to increased satiety after eating, aid weight loss and help lower blood glucose levels.

That mention of fibre near the top of this list.: fibre is good, very good, and I quote from the NHS website:

There is strong evidence that eating plenty of fibre is associated with a lower risk of heart disease, stroke, type 2 diabetes and bowel cancer. Choosing foods with fibre also makes us feel fuller.

And more on ginger: the following is adapted from the Healthline website:

Ginger in any form is an extremely healthy spice, loaded with nutrients and bioactive compounds, benefiting both body and brain function.

It has been used to help digestion, reduce all kinds of nausea and help fight both flu and the common cold. Ginger also has powerful anti-inflammatory and antioxidant effects.

The spice can also reduce muscle pain, improve heart disease risk factors, help treat chronic indigestion and may reduce blood glucose levels and cholesterol. The active ingredient in ginger can help fight infections.

Ginger is one of the very few super foods worthy of the name. What's not to like!

I have personal experience of the anti-inflammatory benefits of ginger when a few doses of the spice magically cured my toothache.

Currently turmeric is also in favour, said to contain many of the same healthy ingredients found in ginger.

Be watchful food

Bread, especially white

White rice and pasta

Potatoes in all forms

Cereals with added sugar. Be aware of 'hidden' sugar in cereals – and bread

Cheese – albeit it has a good protein and calcium content

Butter – spread it thinly on bread and toast

Ice cream

Marmalade – average sugar content 58%

And bananas – an excellent source of potassium, fibre and B6 vitamin, but they also contain more calories and sugar compared to other fruit

Bad food

Hidden sugar in many products – be aware

All processed and refined food

Take-aways, especially Chinese

Pizza

Chips and crisps

Sugar and foods with high sugar content

Salt, and all products with a high salt content

Chocolate

Pineapple, melon, grapes and dates (all full of sugar)

Cakes and biscuits (ditto)

Fruit juices and fizzy drinks (again high in sugar)

Note:

Good food, Be watchful food, Bad food

These are by no means exhaustive lists

11

What a Doctor Suggests

Dr. Mosley – I am one of his biggest fans. I have bought several of his books and have even attended one of his roadshows.

This is the guy who introduced the World to the 5:2 diet, whereby you fast for two days a week and eat normally for the other five; I haven't tried it myself.

All subsequent content in this chapter has been extracted from his books and is to be attributed to him. Some of the content is generic and has been mentioned earlier. So, more repetition, but all worthwhile stuff I believe.

Here we go:

Think very carefully when tempted to buy 'bad'
food (chocolate, chips, crisps etc.)

Chocolate is a classic example of a refined food.
It is the most addictive food, making it hard to
stop after just one piece, and is full of sugar and
fat.

[When I feel I just must satisfy my chocolate
craving, I choose a piece of dark chocolate which
is said to be healthier (but not for dogs,
apparently, for whom it can be fatal). Everyone
deserves the occasional treat]

When glancing at the cake or biscuit tin, look for
a distraction:

Say 'I'll come back to that later'

Go for a walk

Drink water

[The benefits of walking, and drinking water, are
mentioned several times in this book]

Try missing breakfast or lunch occasionally – a
fasting window of 12 daylight hours can be very
effective.

Apparently, Hippocrates recommended fasting

Fasting improves memory

Watch sugar (particularly) and fat in products

Porridge and low sugar muesli are both very good, filling and help reduce cholesterol

To maintain muscle, it is imperative to consume protein, and take exercise

If your body can take it, Dr. Mosley recommends High Intensity Interval Training. This entails building up to 10 x 6-second bursts of activity such as running on the spot. Rest between each burst. Repeat twice weekly. He reckons it can work wonders.

He also says you cannot beat a low carbohydrate diet.

. . . .

This is a very small selection of his thoughts. There's lots more from the good doctor in his numerous books.

12

Diabetes

I refer only to type 2 diabetes (also known as late-onset diabetes). I am not qualified to comment on type 1 diabetes which is in the province of medical professionals.

Those excess pounds can lead to diabetes which in turn can, and does, lead to multiple health issues. A healthy lifestyle is essential to avoid travelling down this road.

A majority of diabetics suffer from high blood pressure and require medication to control both this and their cholesterol.

Diabetics are twice as likely to die from a heart attack and are at increased risk of blindness, kidney disease, dementia and amputations.

A couple of years ago, following a routine blood test, I was told I was 'pre-diabetic', not a diabetic as such but well on my way there.

This scare made it relatively easy for me to make simple changes in my lifestyle, not much more than cutting right back on my three favourite 'baddies' – red wine (ok in moderation but I was over-doing it), cheese and chocolate – and introducing a daily walk into my regime.

Without following a formal diet and with relatively little effort, it took less than three months for me to return to a healthy blood glucose reading. But I have to keep to my amended lifestyle (not always easy) and not fall back into that risky pre-diabetic state.

It is probably not a bad idea to note the common symptoms of type 2 diabetes:

According to the NHS website, these include frequent urination, being thirsty all the time, feeling very tired, losing weight without trying to, blurred vision and cuts or wounds taking longer to heal.

But you don't need to show any of these symptoms to be a diabetic.

13

Heartburn and Related Issues

I suffered these problems for many years until I took action to reverse my pre-diabetic condition.

The changes required in my lifestyle had the added benefit of me being less prone to adverse stomach complaints.

I discovered examples of food that can cause acid reflux: too much fatty food, fizzy drinks, cheese, coffee, alcohol and chocolate – a fairly similar list of products that should be limited if seeking a healthy lifestyle.

Acid reflux and indigestion issues in general are heightened by a large evening meal, particularly if eaten late in the evening. It is generally accepted that we should stop eating three hours before bedtime.

Being overweight aggravates symptoms of discomfort. I am not totally free from indigestion and oesophagus problems but I have far fewer incidences since reducing my weight.

This fell from an excessive 15½ stone (96kg) to a more reasonable 13 stone (82kg) but I am by no means a lightweight. I need to lose a little more.

But my priority is never again to be burdened with those surplus pounds.

I discovered quite recently, and I mention this in case it may be a thought for others, I have an intolerance (I would not say an allergy) to wheat products. I can enjoy a small sandwich or a single slice of toast but any more risks the onset of stomach pain. I get on better with bread containing a reduced wheat content.

Temporary cures for acid reflux, apart from over-the-counter antacid products, include:

An apple

Well-diluted apple cider vinegar (mentioned elsewhere) can help for some

Raw fruit or vegetables, or just plain water

14

High Blood Pressure (Hypertension)

This can be measured at home on a blood pressure monitor, obtainable from any good pharmacy.

If high, say over 150/90, (many GP's now prefer to see a lower reading than this for the middle-aged and elderly, and a lot less for the young), medication can be prescribed.

But readings can be reduced, at least in part, by maintaining a sensible weight and a healthy living regime. Now for an element of more repetition, this time relating to reducing blood pressure:

Exercise regularly

Limit alcohol

Reduce salt intake. Try to stop adding salt to your meals

Keep the salt cellar in the cupboard

No added sugar

Consume good foods as listed in an earlier chapter, particularly fruit and veg, including blueberries and tomatoes; oily fish, low sugar yogurt and even dark chocolate – in moderation.

....

Blood pressure and a general state of health can be affected by stress. I know family and friends who recommend yoga and I understand the benefits but I have as yet to embrace the discipline.

What I have practised is mindfulness.

15

Mindfulness

I do not often suffer from stress but if I have a concern on my mind or particularly find difficulty sleeping, I refer to the following advice:

Close your eyes and imagine a sense of peace, stillness and tranquillity

Rest a moment

Take one long deep breath

Then breathe deeply, but gently

Listen to your breathing

Feel the intake of breath, then slowly exhale

It can help to count up to five breathing in, then up to five breathing out

Let thoughts come and go

Acknowledge distracting thoughts then send them away

Don't dwell on negative feelings, try not to let them take over

Think positive thoughts

Relax all the muscles in your body

Imagine lying on warm soft sand and letting your body relax, sinking into the sand

Think of something pleasant and good in your life

Think contentment.

....

If up and about, go for a stroll and be aware of your surroundings, whether rural or urban. Look at the trees, the buildings, the sky

Listen to the sounds around you

Be mindful of each step you take

When waiting, such as in a queue for a bus or on the telephone, try to avoid agitation and take the moment to rest, to unwind

When eating, eat slowly and think about the food, the flavour, the texture

Try not to worry about what cannot be changed

Focus on the present

A smile is so much better than a frown

Let mindfulness become a foundation for a healthy lifestyle.

. . . .

That is the briefest of summaries. For more thoughts and ideas get hold of one of the numerous books written on the subject.

16

A Dry January

In 2014, 14 members of the *New Scientist*, all of whom considered themselves of 'normal' weight, carried out a study. For a month, ten members drank no alcohol, the others carried on as normal.

Among the ten abstainers, the average level of liver fat had reduced by 15%, blood glucose levels by 23% and they had on average lost 1.5kg in weight. And they all slept better during the trial.

So it's a dry January for me. Well, I'll try...

17

And Finally

I am getting on quite happily with my healthy living and generally eating sensibly. But the demons do try to influence me, telling me how much I would really enjoy a fully-loaded meat feast pizza or a large bag of chips, well salted. I tell them to go away.

I have worked hard at my new lifestyle and am not going to sacrifice what I have achieved so far to return to anything more than occasional comfort eating. No way am I going to throw all that effort away. And this mindful approach works. Usually.

Remember, over-eating is a mindset. If you can train your mind to *really* believe you can change your behaviour, you are well on the way to achieving your goal.

When I face temptations to relapse, I refer back
to chapter 2 in this book and tell myself:

'I am just not that over-eating person anymore,
that's all in the past'

. . . .

A summary the content of this book:

It is important to eat a healthy, balanced diet
generally low in fat, definitely low in sugar and
salt, and high in fruit and vegetables. No surprises
there.

And equally important – keep up the exercise –
a*ny* exercise is better than none.

We know all this but I for one need to be
reminded, constantly.

Finally, in no particular order apart from the first,
I list on the next page my Ten Key Points:

Stop Smoking

Halve alcohol intake (more if you can)

Concentrate on food low in sugar and fat

Avoid highly processed and refined food

No snacking

Five fruit and veg a day (at least)

Occasionally skip a meal

Don't eat if not actually hungry

Eat slowly

And take every opportunity to take exercise

Forward we go together!

. . . .

For optional further reading, I enclose an Appendix giving information on the Glycaemic index

APPENDIX

Glycaemic Index

A knowledge of the glycaemic index (GI) is helpful in relation to healthy living. The following section has been précised and adapted from the NHS website.

. . . .

GI is a rating system for foods containing carbohydrates. It shows how quickly each food affects your blood glucose level when that food is eaten on its own.

Carbohydrate foods that are broken down quickly by your body and cause a rapid increase in blood glucose have a high GI rating and are generally considered Not Good.

High GI foods include:

Sugar and food with a high sugar content

Sugary soft drinks

White bread

White rice

Potatoes in all forms

Low GI foods are broken down more slowly and cause a gradual rise in blood glucose levels over time and include:

Most fruit including apples and pears (but generally not tropical fruit such as pineapple or melon which have a high sugar content)

Vegetables including sweet potato, beans and pulses

Wholegrain foods, such as porridge oats

Some mueslis with no added sugar.

Low GI foods, such as wholegrains, fruit, vegetables, beans and lentils, are foods we should eat regularly as part of a healthy, balanced diet.

However, using the glycaemic index to decide whether foods or combinations of foods are healthy can sometimes be misleading.

Foods with a high GI are not necessarily unhealthy and not all foods with a low GI are healthy. For example, watermelon (GI 72) and parsnips (52) are high GI foods, while chocolate cake (bad) surprisingly has a lower GI value of 38.

Also, foods that contain or are cooked with fat slow down the absorption of carbohydrate, lowering their GI. For example, crisps have a lower GI than potatoes cooked without fat. However, crisps are high in fat and should be eaten in moderation, or best not at all.

If you *only* eat food with a low GI, your diet may become unbalanced.

But as a general rule, low GI foods are good, high GI foods are not.

Low GI foods which cause your blood glucose levels to rise and fall slowly, may help you feel fuller for longer. This could help control your appetite and may be beneficial if you're trying to lose weight.

If you have diabetes, it's useful to understand the glycaemic index because eating food with low GI ratings can help control blood glucose.

But most importantly, research has shown that the ***amount of carbohydrate*** you eat, rather than its GI rating, has the biggest influence on blood glucose levels after meals.

Comprehensive lists of food GI ratings can be found on the Internet and in books covering the subject.

....

ChrisWalker1812@gmail.com